Revitalize Your Shape

Weight Loss Secrets for 40+ Women

Sarah Wellness

Disclosure Statement

Please be aware that the material in this publication is only intended for educational purposes. Every attempt has been made to offer accurate, current, trustworthy, and comprehensive information. Readers understand that the author is not giving out professional or medical advice. This book's information came from a variety of sources.

Table of Contents

Chapter 1: Embracing Change

Introduction: The obstacles and prospects of loss of weight after 40

As we begin on this path towards greater health and vitality, it's critical to know that, as women over 40, we have a particular mix of difficulties and possibilities when it comes to weight reduction. Embracing change is the first step in renewing your form and living a better, more rewarding existence.

The Body's Changing Metabolism

One of the major changes that women face when they hit their 40s is the natural slowdown of metabolism. Metabolism, the

body's process of transforming food into
energy, tends to decline with age.

This implies that the number of calories you burn at rest drops, and it might become tougher to lose weight or maintain your present weight. But don't be dismayed; your metabolism is not your destiny.

While metabolism may slow down, the good news is that with the appropriate technique, you may still reach your weight reduction objectives. By making smart decisions about your nutrition and exercise, you may work with your body, rather than against it, to attain a renewed shape.

Emotional Factors and Self-Acceptance

The route to weight reduction and greater health frequently comes with emotional obstacles. It's typical to deal with self-doubt, body image difficulties, and worries of failure.

Many women over 40 have spent years
raising kids, creating jobs, and supporting
others, sometimes at the sacrifice of their
well-being. It's time to turn the spotlight back
to you, yet this adjustment may be
emotionally draining.

Learning to welcome change entails
understanding these sentiments and building
self-acceptance. Remember that you are
deserving of excellent health and self-care.
Recognize that your value isn't determined by
a number on the scale or your looks.
Your journey is about feeling your best,
inside and out, and your age should never be
a restricting factor.

Setting Realistic Goals

When going on a weight reduction journey beyond 40, it's vital to create realistic, attainable objectives.
Your body is unique, and your journey will be different from anybody else's. The days of crash diets and intensive workout regimes may be behind you, but this is a benefit.

Embrace change by creating reasonable, sustainable objectives. Instead of looking for immediate, short-term achievements, concentrate on long-term health and well-being. This could imply a steady, progressive weight reduction, but it also means creating habits that will serve you for the rest of your life. Remember, it's not only about reducing weight; it's about achieving a better, more fulfilled life.

Your Journey Begins Here

Embracing change is the cornerstone of your weight reduction journey. It means understanding the particular problems you face, loving yourself and your body, and creating realistic objectives that will take you toward a renewed form and a more vibrant future. In the chapters ahead, we will cover the science of weight growth and reduction, diet, exercise, and the emotional components of this transforming journey.

The path may not always be simple, but the benefits are priceless. So, let's take that first step together towards a healthier, happier you, accepting the changes that will characterize your renewed form.

Chapter 2: The Science of Weight Gain and Loss

Recognizing the biology behind variations in weight

Understanding the science behind weight growth and reduction is essential if you're going to transform your body and start a weight loss path that works. You'll be more capable of making wise choices and creating long-term success plans if you comprehend the biological processes that impact your body.

Hormonal Changes and Metabolism

The intricate network of chemical processes known as metabolism takes place in your body to sustain life. It is the process by which food is transformed into energy, which your body needs for everything from physical activity to breathing. As noted in Chapter 1, the natural slowdown of the metabolism is one of the biggest obstacles for women over 40.

There are several explanations for this slowness. First of all, as you become older, you tend to have less muscle mass, and muscle burns more calories at rest than fat. Second, weight gain may be influenced by hormonal changes, namely the decrease in estrogen that occurs during perimenopause and menopause. Your metabolism and fat distribution may be impacted by these hormonal changes.

Knowing your metabolism, however, is about being knowledgeable, not about giving up. With this understanding, you may make decisions that help fend off these changes brought on by aging.

By concentrating on strength training, for instance, you may increase and maintain muscular mass, which can speed up your metabolism. Additionally, by comprehending the function of hormones, you may make dietary and lifestyle choices that will help you reach your weight reduction objectives.

Gaining Fat and Losing Muscle

It has been said that muscle mass is a major factor in the metabolism game. Sarcopenia is the term for the normal aging-related loss of muscle mass. When muscle is lost, your body burns fewer calories when at rest, which may lead to weight gain if your eating habits don't change.

There is some good news, however! Resistance training and strength training may help prevent muscle loss.

These exercises help you maintain or increase your lean muscle mass by promoting muscular development. Improving bone density, balance, and functional fitness, not only raises your metabolic rate but also benefits your general health.

However, the buildup of fat, especially around the waist, tends to grow with age. Known medically as visceral fat, abdominal fat poses a danger for heart disease, diabetes, and certain types of cancer in addition to being an aesthetic issue.
Making healthy decisions and taking action might be sparked by realizing how important it is to reduce visceral fat.

Stress and Sleep's Roles

Your body's capacity to regulate weight is significantly impacted by stress and sleep. Elevated amounts of stress cause the hormone cortisol to be released, which may cause more fat to be stored, especially in the abdomen. Emotional eating and bad food choices may also be caused by long-term stress.

These issues may be made worse by getting too little sleep. Lack of sleep throws off your body's hormonal balance, making you feel more hungry and more drawn to harmful meals. Lack of sleep also impairs your judgment and self-control, making it more difficult to resist temptation.

It gives you the ability to control stress, sleep, and weight gain when you know how these things work together.

You may keep your cortisol levels in check by using stress-reduction techniques like mindfulness, meditation, or deep breathing exercises. It is equally vital to prioritize getting good sleep since it promotes hormone balance and general health.

Knowledge Is Power

As we explore the science of weight growth and reduction, it becomes evident that the first step to overcoming the obstacles presented by aging is comprehending the complex functions of your body. Accept that your weight is influenced by a variety of factors, including hormones, metabolism, muscle mass, stress, and sleep habits. With this knowledge in hand, you'll be more equipped to take charge of your weight reduction efforts and find your way to a more youthful form.

We shall discuss practical applications of this information in the next chapters. We'll discuss diet, physical activity, and methods for stress management and hormone balance. Recall that your decisions, not your age, determine your fate.

Chapter 3: Nutrition and Healthy Eating Habits

Crafting a balanced diet for lasting weight reduction

In your goal to revive your form and begin on a successful weight reduction journey after 40, diet plays a significant part. Crafting a balanced diet that supports your health objectives is not only about what you eat but how you eat and what you understand about your body's shifting demands. In this chapter, we'll study the basics of a sustainable and healthy eating plan.

Nutrient-Rich Foods for Women Over 40

As women age, their bodies need different nutrients to maintain diverse tasks, such as hormone management, bone health, and heart health.

It's crucial to concentrate on nutrient-dense meals that contain the vitamins and minerals required for overall well-being.

Calcium: Calcium is vital for maintaining bone health, particularly for women over 40, since they face an increased risk of osteoporosis. Incorporate dairy products, leafy greens, and fortified meals into your diet.

Vitamin D: Vitamin D is vital for calcium absorption and general health. Exposure to sunshine and meals like fatty fish, egg yolks, and fortified dairy products may help maintain healthy vitamin D levels.

Omega-3 Fatty Acids: These healthy fats boost heart health and may help decrease inflammation. Include fatty fish (such as salmon and mackerel), flaxseeds, chia seeds, and walnuts in your diet.

Fiber: Fiber assists with digestion, increases fullness, and helps manage blood sugar levels. Whole grains, fruits, vegetables, and legumes are good sources of fiber.

Antioxidants: Antioxidants, such as vitamins C and E, may help protect your body from cellular damage. Consume a range of bright fruits and vegetables, such as berries, citrus, and broccoli.

Protein: Protein is necessary for muscle maintenance and general health. Include lean sources of protein including chicken, fish, lean meats, tofu, and beans in your diet.

Hydration: Staying hydrated is vital for every area of your health. Aim for at least eight glasses of water a day, and explore herbal teas or infused water for variation.

Balancing your diet with these nutrient-rich foods will help guarantee that you're satisfying your body's particular demands as a woman over 40.

Portion Control and Mindful Eating

Another crucial part of good eating habits is portion management and mindful eating. As you age, it's natural for your metabolism to slow down, which means your body needs less calories. Portion management helps you manage your calorie intake while still enjoying the foods you love.

Consider these strategies:

- Use smaller plates to limit portion sizes.
- Give attention to hunger and fullness signals.

- To be more mindful of what and how much you are eating, avoid eating in front of the TV or computer.
- Savor your meals, chew carefully, and appreciate the tastes and textures of your food.

Strategies for Managing Cravings

Cravings are a regular difficulty in any weight reduction program. Understanding your urges and how to control them is key to success. Cravings may be induced by different circumstances, including stress, emotions, or dietary deficits.

To handle cravings effectively:

- **Keep a food journal:** Record what you consume and your emotional condition. This may help detect trends and causes for cravings.

- **Stay hydrated:** Dehydration may frequently be misinterpreted as hunger, leading to needless eating.
- **Choose healthier alternatives:** If you're seeking something sweet, go for a piece of fruit. If you're seeking something salty, consider a handful of nuts or seeds.
- **Employ stress management techniques:** Stress might contribute to emotional eating. Engage in activities that help you relax and manage stress, such as yoga, meditation, or deep breathing techniques.

Building Healthy Eating Habits

Crafting a lasting, healthy eating plan is about more than simply what you eat; it's about developing lifetime habits. Avoid crash diets or excessive limitations, since they typically lead to short-term success and long-term discontent.

Instead, concentrate on building a balanced, fun, and practical eating plan that meets your requirements and lifestyle.

In the chapters that follow, we'll go further into particular nutritional recommendations, meal planning, and efficient methods to manage eating out. Remember, your dietary choices are a critical component of your renewed shape journey, and with the appropriate information and habits, you can reach your objectives and keep a healthy you for years to come.

Chapter 4: Exercise and Fitness for EveryBody

Creating a personalized workout regimen for your age and lifestyle

Physical exercise is a cornerstone of every successful weight reduction and regeneration program, particularly for women over 40. But going on a fitness regimen should not be scary; it should be empowering and pleasurable. In this chapter, we will examine the world of exercise and how to design a personalized fitness plan that meets your specific age, body, and lifestyle.

Seeking the Right Exercise for Your Body

First and foremost, it's vital to recognize that there is no one-size-fits-all strategy to exercise.

Your choice of physical activity should coincide with your present fitness level, preferences, and any physical constraints you may have. **Here are some crucial variables to consider:**

Cardiovascular Exercise: Cardio activities like walking, running, cycling, and swimming are fantastic for burning calories and increasing heart health. Choose an activity that you love and can continue over the long run.

Strength Training: Building and maintaining muscular mass is vital for speeding up your metabolism. Strength training might entail lifting weights, utilizing resistance bands, or completing bodyweight exercises like squats and push-ups.

Flexibility and Balance: Yoga and Pilates are fantastic alternatives for developing flexibility, balance, and posture. As we age, these characteristics of fitness become more crucial for avoiding accidents and preserving mobility.

Low-Impact choices: If you have joint concerns or prefer lower-impact exercises, try choices like water aerobics, stationary cycling, or elliptical machines.

Functional Fitness: Functional workouts mirror ordinary actions and may help you keep nimble and competent in your daily life. These exercises frequently include multi-joint motions, such as lunges, squats, and bending.

The trick is to find things that you love and can commit to consistently. Exercise should be a source of joy and empowerment, not a duty.

Strength Training for Women Over 40

As discussed before, maintaining and developing muscle mass is crucial for women over 40. Muscle burns more calories at rest than fat, which implies that boosting your muscle mass may help speed up your metabolism. Strength training also boosts bone density, lowering the incidence of osteoporosis, and improves functional fitness.

When commencing a strength training routine:

Start with small weights or resistance bands to avoid injury and create a foundation.

Focus on complex exercises that train numerous muscular groups, such as squats, deadlifts, and push-ups.
Incorporate both upper and lower body workouts for balanced strength.
Incorporating Flexibility and Balance

As we age, flexibility and balance become critical for preserving mobility and avoiding injury. Activities like yoga and Pilates are perfect for increasing these components of fitness. They not only expand your range of motion but also induce relaxation and relieve tension.

Tips for adding flexibility and balance exercises:

Attend lessons or utilize instructional videos to learn suitable procedures. Aim for a combination of stretching, balancing, and mobility exercises.

Perform these exercises at least a couple of times a week, preferably after your other workouts.

Exercise Safety and Adaptations

Safety is crucial while participating in physical exercise, particularly as we age. **Here are some guidelines to ensure your fitness program is safe and effective:**

Talk to a healthcare professional: Before beginning a new fitness regimen, talk with your healthcare practitioner, particularly if you have any current health concerns.

Warm-up and cool-down: Begin your exercises with a light warm-up to prepare your body for activity and conclude with a cool-down to aid recuperation.

Listen to your body: Pay alert to any indicators of discomfort or pain. It's crucial to discern between regular muscle discomfort and damage.

Change as needed: If you have physical restrictions or health issues, engage with a fitness expert who can help you change workouts to meet your requirements.

Rest and recovery: Adequate rest is vital for avoiding overuse injuries and enabling your body to mend and develop stronger. Aim for at least one or two relaxation days every week.

Incorporating Exercise into Your Lifestyle

One typical challenge to regular exercise is finding the time. Women over 40 generally balance hectic schedules, employment, family, and other commitments.

The secret to success is making exercise a non-negotiable element of your regimen.

Here are ideas to include fitness into your lifestyle:

Set a schedule: Designate particular times for your exercises, just like you would for any other appointment.

Choose activities you enjoy: You're more likely to persist with exercise if you find it fun. Try several hobbies until you find what you enjoy.

Combine family time with fitness: Involve your family in physical activities, such as hiking, bicycling, or playing sports together.

Break it up: If finding time for a continuous workout is tough, try dividing your activity into shorter, more manageable periods throughout the day.

Use technology: There are various fitness apps and online tools that may help you plan exercises and measure your progress.

Setting Realistic Goals

As you commence on your fitness journey, it's crucial to create reasonable and attainable objectives. Aim for a balance between pushing yourself and keeping motivated.

Some frequent fitness objectives for women over 40 may include:

Weight reduction or maintenance: Setting a target for a certain weight or body fat percentage might be motivating.

Strength and muscle gain: Tracking your progress with weightlifting and other strength-based workouts is a great approach to quantify your accomplishment.

Flexibility and balance: Consider objectives linked to better posture, balance, and flexibility, which may have a substantial influence on everyday living.

Cardiovascular fitness: Monitor your progress with cardiovascular activities by recording your endurance and the distances you can cover.

Adapting to Your Age and Lifestyle

As a woman over 40, it's crucial to modify your fitness program to your age and lifestyle.

Consider these factors:

Rest and recovery: Give your body ample time to recuperate between exercises, particularly if you're new to fitness or escalating your program.

Hormone swings: Be mindful of how your hormone variations may impact your energy levels and emotions. Modify your exercises appropriately.

Joint health: If you have joint difficulties or discomfort, opt for lower-impact workouts and speak with a healthcare practitioner or physical therapist for help.

Balancing family and work: Prioritize self-care and exercise as a technique to manage stress and preserve your general health.

Conclusion: Empowering Your Fitness Journey

Creating a specific workout regimen for your age and lifestyle is an empowering step on your way to a renewed form. Remember that exercise should be a pleasant and fun component of your life, not a punishment or necessity. Choose things that you enjoy, establish reasonable objectives, and tailor your exercises to your particular requirements. In the chapters that follow, we will look into ways to control stress, enhance sleep, and seek support on your rejuvenation journey. You can influence your destiny, and fitness is a critical tool on that transforming road.

Chapter 5: Mind Over Matter: Emotional Eating and Stress Management

Exploring the psychological factors of weight loss

As we continue our path toward renewing our bodies it's critical to realize the enormous influence that emotions and stress can have on your eating patterns and general well-being.

In this chapter, we'll dig into the realm of emotional eating, stress management, and how regulating your emotions may play a vital part in attaining sustained weight loss success.

The Connection Between Eating and Emotions

Emotional eating is a frequent practice that many individuals indulge in at some time in their lives. It's the act of eating in reaction to emotions, such as stress, grief, boredom, or even happiness. For women over 40, the pressures of life, including friends and family, profession, and private ambitions, may cause emotional eating.

Here's why recognizing this link is crucial:

Emotional eating regularly requires eating high-calorie, low-nutrient items, which may hinder your weight reduction objectives. This habit may lead to a cycle of guilt, since you may feel regretful or dissatisfied after giving in to emotional eating.
Emotional eating, contrarily, can be a technique to mask or hide feelings, however, it does not deal with the root causes.

To combat emotional eating, it's crucial to understand the factors that influence it and establish alternate coping mechanisms. Start by maintaining a food and mood diary to detect trends and emotional triggers connected to your eating habits.

Stress Management Techniques

Stress is an inherent aspect of life, and how you handle it may dramatically affect your weight reduction journey. Chronic stress may lead to many mental and physical difficulties, including obesity and emotional eating. Therefore, it's vital to acquire efficient stress management skills.

Consider the following ways to handle stress effectively:

Mindfulness & Meditation: These techniques help you remain present in the moment and lessen worry. You might start with brief, daily mindfulness exercises or guided meditation sessions.

Deep Breathing: Deep, leisurely breathing may assist in relaxing your nervous system and lessen tension. Try to include deep breathing exercises in your routine.

Exercise: Physical exercise, such as walking, running, or yoga, may produce endorphins, which are natural mood boosters. Regular exercise is another way to manage stress and cut emotional eating.

Journaling: Keeping a diary may be a therapeutic approach to expressing your sentiments and reflecting on your emotions. It might give insight into your concerns and help you discover solutions.

Time Management: Learning to prioritize and manage your time properly helps alleviate stress caused by feeling overloaded with chores and obligations.

Social Support: Share your emotions with friends or family members who can give emotional support. Engaging with other individuals can potentially lower stress and emotional eating.

Professional assistance: If your stress is intense and persistent, consider obtaining assistance from a therapist or counselor who specializes in stress management and emotional well-being.

Self-Care and Self-Compassion

In your path toward weight loss and revitalization, it's necessary to practice self-care and self-compassion. Self-compassion entails treating oneself with care and empathy, particularly in periods of conflict or difficulty. Ultimately might be a vital aid in overcoming the addiction of emotional eating and managing stress.

Here are some self-compassion strategies to consider:

Positive Self-Talk: Replace self-criticism with positive and self-affirming beliefs. Treat yourself like you would a dear friend in hard circumstances.

Self-Care Rituals: Engage in self-care activities that feed your body and mind, such as taking a warm bath, reading a good book, or practicing a hobby.

Set Realistic Expectations: Understand that no one is flawless, and failures are a part of every path.

Instead of concentrating on failures, concentrate on what you've learned and the progress you've achieved.

Gratitude: Regularly practice gratitude by thinking about the wonderful things in your life. Gratitude might help shift your interest away from stress and emotional eating triggers.

Overcoming the vicious circle of Emotional Eating

Breaking the pattern of emotional eating is a crucial step toward accomplishing your weight reduction and regeneration objectives.

To accomplish this, it is important to:

Diagnose emotional triggers: Understand the feelings or activities that encourage emotional eating. Keep a diary to help you monitor these triggers.

Develop alternate coping strategies: Instead of resorting to food, develop healthy methods to handle your emotions. Engage in stress-reducing activities or chat with someone you trust.

Employ an expert aid if necessary: If emotional eating is deeply established and tough to manage on your own, find help from a consultant or therapist who makes a specialty in emotional eating.
Remember that this path is about more than simply physical change; it's about emotional and mental well-being as well.

As you control your emotions and learn healthy methods to deal with stress, you'll be more able to reach your weight reduction and rejuvenation objectives. In the chapters that follow, we'll examine the significance of sleep and hormonal balance in your transforming path.

Chapter 6: Sleep, Hormones, and Weight Loss

Understanding the vital role of sleep in weight management

The link between sleep, hormones, and weight control is a fascinating and frequently unappreciated element of the weight reduction process. In this chapter, we will investigate the subtle relationships between these aspects and find how prioritizing sleep and hormonal balance may substantially affect your attempts to renew your form.

The Influence of Sleep on Hormone Regulation

Sleep is a vital biological activity that plays a critical function in regulating numerous hormones inside your body.

Hormones are chemical messengers that influence several body activities, including metabolism, hunger, and stress response. When sleep is interrupted or insufficient, it may lead to hormone imbalances that influence your weight and general health.

Leptin and Ghrelin: The Hunger Hormones

Two major hormones that directly regulate hunger and eating behavior are leptin and ghrelin.

Leptin: Often referred to as the "satiety hormone," leptin is produced by your fat cells and communicates to your brain that you're full and have enough energy. Adequate sleep helps maintain appropriate leptin levels, lowering feelings of hunger and the chance of overeating.

Ghrelin: Ghrelin is known as the "hunger hormone" because it increases appetite and encourages the consumption of food. When you don't get enough sleep, ghrelin levels rise, leading to increased appetite and cravings, especially for high-calorie, carbohydrate-rich meals.

Inadequate or poor-quality sleep may disturb the balance of these hormones, making it hard to regulate your appetite and make appropriate eating choices.

Insulin and Blood Sugar Control

Proper sleep is also crucial for controlling insulin, a hormone that plays a major role in blood sugar regulation. When you're sleep-deprived, your body gets insensitive to insulin, resulting in higher blood sugar levels and an increased chance of developing insulin resistance and type 2 diabetes.

Unstable blood sugar may also drive sugar cravings, making it difficult to keep to a balanced diet.

Cortisol: The Stress Hormone

Cortisol, generally referred to as the "stress hormone," has a varied function in weight regulation. It may be advantageous in acute stress conditions, giving the body a burst of energy to react to a danger. However, persistent stress and poor sleep may lead to high cortisol levels, which have various detrimental consequences for weight and health:

Increased hunger: High cortisol levels may boost your appetite, especially for high-sugar, high-fat meals.

Fat storage: Cortisol stimulates fat storage, especially in the abdominal area, leading to an increased risk of visceral fat buildup.

Muscular loss: Elevated cortisol levels may contribute to muscular breakdown, which can impair your metabolic rate.

Strategies for Improving Sleep

Given the vital function of sleep in hormone control and weight management, it's crucial to emphasize excellent sleep hygiene.

Here are some techniques to help you attain restorative sleep:

Establish a consistent sleep schedule: Try to go to bed and get up at the same time every day, especially on weekends.

Create a peaceful nighttime routine:
Engage in calming activities before bed, such as reading, having a warm bath, or practicing relaxation methods like deep breathing.

Ensure a good sleep environment: Make your bedroom favorable to sleep by keeping it dark, cool, and quiet.

Limit screen time: Avoid electronic gadgets like smartphones and tablets before bedtime, since the blue light produced might interfere with sleep.

Watch your caffeine intake: Avoid caffeine in the afternoon and evening, since it might alter sleep patterns.

Mind your diet: Heavy or spicy meals close to bedtime might lead to indigestion and impair sleep. Plan to finish eating no sooner than two to three hours before bedtime.

Exercise regularly: Engaging in physical activity may enhance sleep quality, but avoid severe exercise close to bedtime.

Hormonal Balance and Managing Weight

Achieving hormonal balance is a challenging but crucial component of good weight control. Here are some other techniques to help hormonal balance and weight loss:

Manage stress: Incorporate stress management practices, such as meditation, deep breathing, or yoga, into your daily routine to help control cortisol levels.

Stay hydrated: Proper hydration helps hormone regulation. Aim to drink enough water throughout the day.

Eat a balanced diet: Consume nutrient-dense foods that promote hormone balance, such as whole grains, lean proteins, and a range of fruits and vegetables.

Limit processed meals and added sugars: Highly processed foods and excessive sugar consumption may alter hormone balance. Lower your consumption of such foods.

See a healthcare professional: If you feel hormone abnormalities are influencing your weight control, see a healthcare practitioner who can do the necessary tests and give advice.

Conclusion: The Power of Quality Sleep and Hormonal Harmony

Sleep and hormonal balance are two frequently ignored yet powerful instruments on your road to renewing your form.

By emphasizing enough quality sleep and maintaining hormonal equilibrium, you may boost your appetite management, improve blood sugar control, and handle stress more efficiently.

In the chapters that follow, we'll discuss the significance of support networks, accountability, and success stories to motivate and lead you on your road to a healthier, reinvigorated self. Remember that the journey is not only about reducing weight; it's about embracing a better, more vibrant future.

Chapter 7: Support Systems and Accountability

Building a network for success

As you continue your path toward renewing your body and accomplishing your weight reduction objectives, you'll discover that having a solid support system and a feeling of responsibility may be important in remaining on track. In this chapter, we will dig into the relevance of these variables and investigate how they may help you achieve sustainable success.

The Importance of Social Support

When you begin a weight reduction and rejuvenation journey, it's necessary to have a network of support from friends, family, or even other persons with similar aims.

The Advantages of social support are numerous:

Motivation: Knowing that people believe in you and your endeavor may be tremendously inspiring. The encouragement and positive reinforcement from your support system may keep you on track, even when things are rough.

Accountability: When you have people who are aware of your objectives and progress, you're more likely to remain committed. Accountability to someone else may be a tremendous motivation in accomplishing your aims.

Emotional support: Weight reduction may be an emotional process, packed with highs and lows. Having someone to speak to or depend on during hard times may give comfort and understanding.

Practical Assistance: Support from friends or family may extend to practical assistance, such as help with food preparation, babysitting, or giving chances for physical exercise.

Healthy rivalry: In certain circumstances, friendly competition with individuals who share similar objectives may be a pleasant and encouraging approach to keeping on track.

Building Your Support System

To construct a solid support system, consider the following steps:

Share Your Goals: Communicate your weight loss and rejuvenation objectives with individuals you trust. Explain why these objectives are crucial to you and how they may assist your efforts.

Seek Like-Minded Individuals: Join weight loss or fitness organizations, either in person or online, to interact with people who have similar objectives. These networks may give useful guidance, inspiration, and accountability.

Enlist a Workout Buddy: Find a friend or family member who shares your passion for fitness. Having a workout buddy may make exercising more fun and generate a feeling of responsibility.

Engage with specialists: Consider obtaining help from specialists, such as a qualified nutritionist, personal trainer, or therapist. Their knowledge may give essential help and direction.

Use Technology: Utilize fitness apps, online forums, or social media platforms to interact with like-minded folks and measure your progress.

Setting Up an Accountability System

While social support may give emotional and motivational advantages, an accountability system adds an organized, goal-focused component to your path.

Here are some techniques for generating accountability:

Set Clear, Measurable Objectives: Your objectives should be precise, measurable, attainable, relevant, and time-bound (SMART). These traits make it easy to measure your development.

Regular Progress Tracking: Keep a record of your food consumption, activity, and weight changes. Utilize a notebook, smartphone app, or even a spreadsheet to chronicle your progress.

Create a Rewards System: Develop a rewards system to commemorate milestones and triumphs. Rewards may provide positive reinforcement for your hard effort.

Share Your Goals and Progress: Share your goals and progress with your support system and ask for their engagement in your accountability efforts. They may check in on your progress often and give comments.

Consider Professional Accountability: Engage with a healthcare practitioner, personal trainer, or nutritionist who can give organized accountability and direction.

Accountability Partners: Connect with an accountability partner who shares similar aims. Regular check-ins, whether in person or digitally, may help you remain on target.

Overcoming Challenges with Accountability

While accountability may be incredibly beneficial, it's necessary to approach it with a balanced viewpoint. Here are a few ideas for solving frequent challenges:

Stay Flexible: Life may be unexpected. If you skip a workout or eat an excessive meal, don't consider it a failure. Instead, alter your strategy and continue ahead.

Learn from Setbacks: If you meet barriers or plateaus, consider them as chances to learn and adapt your strategy. It's common to confront hurdles on your trip.

Regularly examine and Adjust objectives:
Periodically examine your objectives and
progress. If required, alter your objectives to
ensure they stay reasonable and attainable.

Maintain Self-Compassion: Be gentle and
patient with yourself. Weight reduction is not
a linear process, and setbacks are a normal
part of the road.

Celebrate Triumphs: Don't forget to
appreciate and celebrate your triumphs, no
matter how minor. Celebrating milestones
helps keep you motivated and focused on
your ultimate objective.

Conclusion: The Power of Support and Accountability

A solid support system and a structured
accountability system may be game-changers

in your weight reduction and regeneration journey. They give the incentive, emotional support, and disciplined monitoring essential to remain on track and achieve permanent success.

In the chapters that follow, we will examine real-life success stories and practical recommendations to inspire and lead you in your transforming path. Remember, you have the power to influence your future, and the correct support and accountability may help you reach your objectives.

Chapter 8: Success Stories and Real-Life Transformations

Inspiration and understanding from those who have been there

In the quest for weight reduction and rejuvenation, few things are as inspirational and educational as the real-life success stories of people who have overcome hurdles, improved their lives, and accomplished their health and fitness objectives. In this chapter, we will study amazing success stories and garner useful ideas from others who've walked the same journey you're on today.

The Power of Real-Life Success Stories

Success stories are not only reports of physical transformation; they are tales of persistence, tenacity, and unrelenting dedication to change. They give hope and indicate that big changes are achievable, regardless of the barriers encountered. Success stories are a source of motivation and encouragement for anybody beginning a weight reduction and rejuvenation journey.

Meet Sarah: Overcoming Health Challenges

Sarah's adventure started when she was confronted with a series of health difficulties. She had high blood pressure, was pre-diabetic, and her doctor had voiced worries about her weight. These medical difficulties were her wake-up call.

Sarah's Insights:

Seek Professional Guidance: Sarah visited a healthcare physician and certified nutritionist to design a tailored weight reduction and health improvement strategy. Professional counsel may be beneficial.

Start Moderate: Instead of making huge adjustments, Sarah started with moderate, sustainable improvements to her diet and exercise regimen. This helped her to form enduring habits.

Stay Consistent: Sarah highlighted the significance of consistency. Weight reduction and health changes take time, and progress may be sluggish. The trick is to keep going.

Meet James: Embracing a Lifestyle Change

James's path entailed a considerable lifestyle transformation. He had a sedentary profession and was used to bad eating habits. To reform his life, he needed to modify not just what he ate but how he lived.

James's Insights:

Plan Your Meals: James learned the significance of food planning. This helped him make better dietary choices and prevent hasty selections.

Incorporate Physical Exercise: He introduced physical exercise into his regular regimen. Initially, this meant taking small walks during work breaks and gradually increasing his exercise level.

Lean on Support: James underlined the significance of a support system. His wife accompanied him on his adventure, which offered incentive, accountability, and friendship.

Meet Maria: A Shift in Mindset

For Maria, the path to weight reduction and rejuvenation was not only about physical changes; it was also about transforming her thinking and relationship with food. Her previous regimen was plagued with emotive eating, and she had to address the emotional aspects of her journey.

Maria's Insights:

Embrace Self-Care: Maria learned to emphasize self-care, including mindfulness and stress management. These strategies helped her handle emotional eating triggers.

Mindful Eating: She embraced mindful eating strategies, which helped her to pay attention to hunger and fullness signals and make wiser meal choices.

Set Realistic Objectives: Maria discovered that creating modest, realistic objectives was crucial to her success. These objectives gave frequent victories and encouragement.

A Common Thread: Resilience and Patience

One common thread throughout these success tales is persistence and patience. Weight reduction and regeneration are not linear paths. Setbacks are normal, and the route may be tough. However, each of these people fought hurdles with persistence, adapted to their surroundings, and stayed patient throughout their changes.

Guidance for Your Journey

While each person's path is unique, there are certain common concepts and tactics that you may use for your own weight reduction and rejuvenation journey:

Start with a Clear Why: Understand your motives for beginning on this trip. Your "why" will give inspiration throughout challenging times.

Seek Professional Guidance: Consider speaking with a healthcare physician, certified nutritionist, or personal trainer who can help you design a tailored strategy.

Set Realistic Objectives: Create objectives that are precise, measurable, realistic, relevant, and time-bound (SMART). This ensures that your goals are clear and reachable.

Be Consistent: Consistency is indispensable. Make healthful practices a part of your everyday routine.

Use Support and Accountability: Lean on your support system, and consider developing an accountability system to measure your progress.

Prioritize Self-Care: Pay attention to your emotional and mental well-being. Develop self-care techniques, such as mindfulness and stress management.

Learn from Setbacks: When setbacks arise, consider them as chances to learn and adapt your approach.

Celebrate Successes: Acknowledge and celebrate every milestone, no matter how minor. This will keep you motivated and focused on your final objective.

Conclusion: Your Success Story Awaits

The remarkable success stories and lessons presented here serve as a monument to the transformational power of drive, perseverance, and a commitment to change. By embracing the knowledge and experiences of people who have traveled the route before you, you may discover inspiration, motivation, and essential direction for your own weight reduction and rejuvenation journey.

In the chapters that follow, we will cover practical ways to preserve your success and incorporate these new habits into your long-term lifestyle. Remember that you can control your destiny, and your success narrative is ready to be written.

Chapter 9: Staying on Track: Maintenance and Beyond

Ensuring long-term prosperity and a bright future

As you reach the last chapters of your weight loss and rejuvenation journey, it's necessary to contemplate what happens next. Maintenance is a vital step that will decide the long-term effectiveness of your change.

In this chapter, we will cover ways to keep on track, retain your success, and embrace a bright and healthy future.

The Challenge of Weight Maintenance

Weight reduction is a remarkable feat, but sustaining your achievements may be just as tough, if not more so. Many people who find early success may confront the issue of regaining lost weight. The causes behind this might vary but generally include a return to previous behaviors and a lack of continued drive.

However, with the correct tactics and mentality, you may traverse the maintenance period effectively and experience lasting effects.

Embracing Lifestyle Changes

The cornerstone of weight maintenance is found in lifestyle modifications. The behaviors you've formed during your trip need to become a permanent part of your everyday life.

This doesn't mean you can never enjoy a particular treat or miss a workout, but it does imply that generally, you emphasize a healthy and balanced lifestyle.

Consistency is Key

Consistency is key in the maintenance phase. Continue to:

Monitor your progress: Regularly weigh yourself or check your measurements to notice any symptoms of weight gain early.

Keep a watch on your diet: Pay attention to your eating habits and ensure they stay connected with your objectives.

Stay active: Maintain a regular workout plan that you love and that fits into your lifestyle.

Prioritize self-care: Continue to manage stress and concentrate on your emotional well-being. This can help you prevent emotional eating and disappointments.

The Role of Accountability

Accountability might be even more crucial during the maintenance period. While you may no longer require the same degree of support as during your first weight reduction journey, any type of accountability will help you remain on track.

Consider these strategies:

Regular check-ins: Continue to have regular accountability check-ins with a friend, family member, or support group.

Set new goals: Define fresh health and exercise objectives to keep your motivation strong. This may be striving for a new fitness milestone, learning a new physical activity, or adjusting your nutrition.

Enjoy milestones: As you maintain your weight, recognize and enjoy your accomplishment, even if it means maintaining your present weight without additional reduction.

Accountability partners: Lean on an accountability partner or group that shares your upkeep objectives and problems.

Maintaining Your Mindset

Your thinking plays a key part in the maintenance phase. Remember that this journey is not only about reducing weight; it's about establishing a healthier and more vibrant future. To preserve your results, it's vital to:

Remain Adaptable: Be prepared to make changes when life throws curveballs. If you meet setbacks, concentrate on resilience and adaptation.

Stress Management: Focus on stress management to avoid emotional eating and other stress-related difficulties.

Focus on self-care: Your emotional and mental well-being should remain a priority. Engage in mindfulness and relaxation practices to help your overall wellness.

Long-Term Goals

Your weight maintenance journey should not be considered as the conclusion of your transformation but as a stepping stone to long-term health and energy. While the original emphasis may have been on weight reduction, adjust your viewpoint toward enjoying a bright and active future.

Consider these long-term goals:

Ideal health: Strive for ideal physical and mental health. This involves maintaining good blood pressure, blood sugar levels, and cholesterol, as well as a robust immune system.

Active living: Continue to live an active lifestyle that incorporates frequent exercise and physical activities that you love.

Balanced nutrition: Maintain a balanced and healthy diet that promotes your overall health and energy levels.

Emotional Well-being: Focus on your emotional well-being, creating a happy and resilient mentality.

Quality of life: The ultimate objective is to experience a great quality of life, full of vitality, excitement, and a vivid future.

Conclusion: A Vibrant and Healthy Future

Your weight reduction and rejuvenation journey is a testimonial to your dedication, tenacity, and persistence. As you move into the maintenance phase and beyond, remember that this is not the end of your transformation; it's the beginning of a bright and healthy future.

In the last chapter, we will examine the enduring impact of your narrative and how it

might inspire and assist others on their road
to a better and rejuvenated life.

You can determine your destiny, and your narrative may be a source of inspiration and encouragement for others around you.

Chapter 10: Your Roadmap to a Revitalized Shape

Empowering your path to permanent change

In this last chapter, you'll take the ideas, tactics, and inspiration gained during your weight reduction and rejuvenation journey and build your unique path to a reinvigorated form. This roadmap will serve as your guide to sustaining your successes and embracing a future filled with health, energy, and enduring well-being.

Reflecting on Your Journey

Before we construct your unique roadmap, take time to think about the trip you've begun. Remember the early motives, struggles, and triumphs that have taken you to this point.

Acknowledge the hard work, dedication, and personal development you've achieved along the road.

Your Roadmap

Your customized roadmap is a dynamic strategy that adjusts to your developing requirements and ambitions. It involves your physical, emotional, and mental well-being, ensuring that your change extends to all parts of your life.

Step 1: Define Your Long-Term Goals

Your first step is to determine your long-term objectives. These should include all elements of your life, including physical, emotional, and mental wellness. Consider the following questions:

Physical Health: What health objectives do you wish to achieve? These can include maintaining your weight, increasing your fitness, or obtaining certain health indicators like blood pressure and cholesterol levels.

Emotional Well-Being: How do you wish to feel emotionally and mentally? Do you wish to minimize stress, develop your emotional resilience, or improve your general mental health?

Quality of Life: What does a high-quality life mean to you? What interests, hobbies, or experiences do you wish to embrace?

Step 2: Create SMART Goals

With your long-term objectives in mind, set SMART (Specific, Measurable, Achievable, Relevant, Time-bound) targets. SMART goals give clear guidance and guarantee that your objectives are reasonable and achievable.

Specific: Define the particular details of your aim. For example, if you aim to maintain your weight, select your desired weight range.

Measurable: Use measurable measurements to monitor your development. If you wish to enhance your fitness, select the number of exercises or your exercise time.

Achievable: Ensure that your objectives are practical and within grasp. Setting excessively ambitious objectives might lead to frustration.

Relevant: Make sure your goals match your long-term aims and beliefs. For instance, if you aim to minimize stress, specify particular stress management practices you will apply.

Time-bound: Set a specific deadline for attaining your objectives. Having a deadline generates a feeling of urgency and helps you monitor your progress.

Step 3: Develop a Sustainable Plan

Your strategy should incorporate your diet, exercise, stress management, and self-care routines. Ensure that your strategy is sustainable, pleasant, and adaptable to varied life conditions.
Here are crucial considerations for each part of your plan:

Nutrition: Maintain a balanced and healthy diet that promotes your long-term health. Continue to practice mindful eating, watch your quantities, and pay attention to the quality of your food choices.

Workout: Continue with a regular workout plan that you love. Mix up your activities to keep things new and intriguing. Stay consistent and change your routines as your fitness level improves.

Stress Management: Incorporate stress management practices into your everyday life. This may involve meditation, deep breathing, or regular mindfulness practices.

Self-Care: Prioritize self-care and emotional well-being. Engage in things that offer you pleasure and relaxation, and seek help when required.

Step 4: Build and Maintain Accountability

Accountability is a strong tool for remaining on track. Set up a strategy that holds you responsible for your objectives and success. Consider the following options:

Accountability Partner: Continue to work with an accountability partner who shares your objectives and can give support and encouragement.

Regular Check-Ins: Schedule regular check-ins with yourself to analyze your progress, change your strategy, and celebrate your triumphs.

Support Groups: Join or continue engaging in support groups, whether in person or online. These communities may give useful insight and inspiration.

Professional Guidance: If required, contact healthcare experts, such as registered dietitians, personal trainers, or therapists, who may give continuous support and expertise.

Step 5: Embrace a Resilient Mindset

Your mentality is a key component of your path. Cultivate a resilient attitude that incorporates the following principles:

Adaptability: Be prepared to adjust to life's changes and difficulties. Life is full of unexpected turns, and the capacity to adapt is a key to success.

Self-Compassion: Practice self-compassion and kindness to oneself. Treat yourself like you would a dear friend when setbacks arise.

Appreciate triumphs: Acknowledge and appreciate your triumphs, no matter how minor. One powerful motivator is positive reinforcement.

Continuous Learning: View setbacks and obstacles as chances for development and learning. They are a natural part of your path.

Step 6: Share Your Story and Inspire Others

Your journey is a tremendous narrative of development and resilience. Consider sharing your experiences with others to encourage and help them on their journey to revival. Your experience might be a source of encouragement and hope for people who may be experiencing similar struggles.

Conclusion: A Vibrant and Enduring Future

Your roadmap to a rejuvenated form is a live document, adapted to your shifting requirements and ambitions. As you go on in your path, remember that this is not the end but the beginning of a lively and lasting future.

Your transformation is a monument to your perseverance, resilience, and steadfast commitment to change. The obstacles you've faced, the habits you've formed, and the progress you've experienced have enabled you to embrace a healthier, more vibrant future.

Your story is an inspiration, not only for yourself but for everyone around you. By sharing your experience and the insights you've received, you may lead others on their road to revival.

You can change your destiny, and your narrative is a light of hope and encouragement for others.

Final Thoughts: Your Rejuvenated Future

As you come to the end of your life-changing adventure toward a renewed future, pause to consider the incredible distance you have traveled. Along with losing extra weight, you've also welcomed a feeling of improved health, energy, and well-being. Your narrative demonstrates your dedication, fortitude, and unrelenting will to build a better, healthier future.

Your path has been a dynamic one, full of obstacles and victories, failures and accomplishments. Through it all, you have developed the habits required for long-lasting transformation, found your inner strength, and understood the value of having a resilient attitude.

However, this is only the start of an endlessly rejuvenated future—not the end. Your reenergized future is a colorful tapestry of health, pleasure, and a life well-lived, not simply a series of numbers on a scale.

Accepting Physical Wellness: The state of optimum health you've attained defines your rejuvenated future. You've made it possible for your life to be unrestricted by issues with blood sugar, hypertension, or ill health. You have the skills and habits necessary to look for your physical health today.

Developing Mental and Emotional Resilience: In your reenergized future, mental and emotional health are paramount. You've mastered stress management and self-care prioritization, which equips you to overcome obstacles in life with fortitude and optimism.

Quality of Existence: You have a high-quality existence in your rejuvenated future. You possess the vitality, vigor, and excitement necessary to seize every opportunity, follow your interests, realize your aspirations, and make enduring memories with those you love.

Telling Your Story: Your story has immense power. You help and encourage others on their roads to revival by sharing your experience. Your narrative serves as a source of inspiration, a ray of hope, and evidence of the capacity for transformation that exists within each of us.

Your Roadmap: Your roadmap is your compass for the path ahead, full of SMART objectives, resilience, and the force of responsibility. It will change with you, according to your ever-shifting requirements and goals.

The Future Is Yours: There are many opportunities in this reinvigorated future. You can write the story of your own life and design a well-lived, happy, and long-lasting existence. The obstacles you've surmounted and the knowledge you've acquired are your instruments for creating a more promising and healthful future.

Your renewed future is an ode to your fortitude, resiliency, and willingness to adapt. It's an endless future filled with all the vitality, health, and happiness you've worked so hard to achieve.

Always keep in mind that your tale is one of strength and inspiration as you continue to carve out your renewed future.

The journey is about a deep change in your whole life, not simply about losing weight. With wide arms and a resolute faith in the lasting power of your rejuvenated self, welcome the future.